A Leptin Mediterranean Diet

Exploration Over 50 Enticing Recipes To Energise Your Day and Excite Your Palate

By: Emily Simmons

While every precaution has been taken in the preparation of this book, the publisher assumes no responsibility for errors or omissions, or for damages resulting from the use of the information contained herein.

A LEPTIN MEDITERRANEAN DIET EXPLORATION OVER 50 ENTICING RECIPES TO ENERGISE YOUR DAY AND EXCITE YOUR PALATE

First edition. June 23, 2021.

ISBN: 979-8201577476

Written by Emily Simmons.

Table of contents

INTRODUCTION

Introduction

So, what exactly is "Leptin-Mediterranean" anyway?

Leptin is a little molecule, a hormone actually, that is responsible for controlling fat storage in our bodies. It controls which nutrients get stored as fat, and which are going to be directly used for energy. In obese people, leptin is usually in short supply, so their bodies need a nudge to produce the correct levels. Studies have shown that this "nudge" can be provided by 5 basic things:

1. Not eating after an early dinner. (Eating late causes almost every calorie consumed to be stored as fat.)
2. Eating 3 meals a day without snacking in between. The idea is to maintain 3-6 hours between meals without having other food as well. We often perceive thirst in between meals as hunger, so rather than snack, drink plenty of water.
3. Don't eat big meals. It's a misconception that people in Mediterranean regions eat huge dishes full of pasta and meat, with big wedges of bread on the side, along with bottle after bottle of red wine. In truth, they have several small dishes, consisting mainly of fruit and vegetables with some legumes, and small amounts of meat as flavoring, with a glass of wine. But more about that just now. If our bodies are fed large amounts of food in one go, we can be sure that some of it will be stored as fat. Large meals interfere with the production of leptins by our bodies.

1. Eat a protein-rich breakfast, focusing on breakfast as the main meal of the day, rather than dinner. There's an old saying that has some wisdom, "Eat breakfast like a king, lunch like a peasant, and supper like a pauper." So, you'll find our breakfast recipes here are full of good proteins like lean ham, eggs, feta cheese, chicken breast, and lean beef. Try them, and you'll eliminate those mid-morning hunger pangs.

2. Reduce (don't eliminate) the amount of carbohydrates eaten. Our bodies are designed to crave them for times of survival, in order to increase fat reserves, which is exactly what we don't need in these times of relative abundance. Rather fill up on fruits, vegetables, cottage cheese, yoghurts, or make some delicious healthy soups from our soup chapter.

As far as Mediterranean food goes,
it is essentially balanced between the sea and the
land.

I say, "From the land," because of the gorgeous olive oils, honey, nuts, vegetables, fruits, meats, and legumes that are produced; "From the sea," because the cuisine incorporates good amounts of fish and shellfish. Dishes from the Mediterranean region normally retain an essential freshness and simplicity. Food here is always more than just nourishment for the body. It is also nourishment for the soul, for family bonds, and for friendship. Even in these modern days of busyness and rush, time is still taken in the preparation of the food and the enjoyment of it. The principle of "slow food", which has become so trendy in the West, has been practiced for centuries in the Mediterranean region.

Staples in the region's kitchens are wheat (made into flour for pastas, breads, and pastries); vegetables (notably tomatoes, artichokes, courgettes, peppers, garlic, among many others); legumes (dried beans, lentils, chickpeas); and, of course, herbs and spices for flavoring all of this ((pepper, thyme, rosemary, bay, cumin, nutmeg, cinnamon etc.) Oils, too, are a staple, particularly olive. Meats are lean and are secondary to the meal- more of a flavoring than a base for the whole dish. Sweets are usually fruits, such as figs, grapes, and oranges, with the odd pastry as well. There is an emphasis on fresh, homegrown, or homemade produce, rather than processed food.

The benefits of eating this way have been known about and studied since after the Second World War, when studies were done comparing the cardio-vascular health and longevity of men in the West and those in the Mediterranean lands.

So, what we've done in this book is combine the modern principles that are known of leptin's role in weight control, with the ancient way of eating that has been practiced for centuries in the Mediterranean region that is known to promote health, and we've come up with some simple, healthy, and delicious recipes that we hope will become part of your everyday diet. So, if you want protection against type 2 diabetes, heart disease and stroke; a reduced risk of developing Alzheimer's; a decreased risk of getting Parkinson's disease; increased longevity, as well as a day filled with delicious easy-to-cook meals, then make this recipe book a part of your lifestyle!

LEPTIN-MEDITERRANEAN HEALTHY BREAKFAST RECIPES

So, let's begin at sunrise. A great breakfast is where a day full of energy begins, and where you start to beat those mid-morning hunger pangs. You should notice improved concentration for your work morning, too. We've given you a selection of quick-to-make recipes for busy weekday mornings, as well as some for the weekend when you have a little more time.

Mediterranean Ham and Egg Cups

This one's full of good things, like spinach and feta, as well as a good dose of protein from the eggs. Basil and pesto add flavour and freshness.

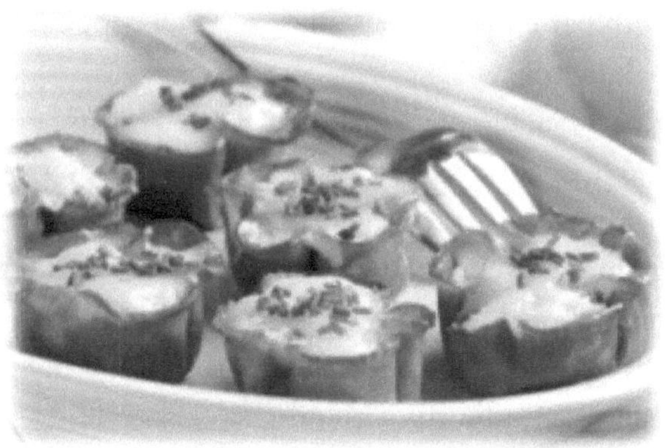

SERVES: 6

INGREDIENTS:

- 6 slices of thin cut deli ham
- 1 large red bell pepper, roasted, peeled and seeded, quartered
- 1/3 cup fresh spinach, finely chopped

- 1/4 cup low-fat feta cheese, crumbled
- 8 egg whites
- 1 large whole egg
- Salt and freshly ground black pepper, to taste
- 2 tablespoons of pesto sauce
- Oil, for greasing muffin tin
- Fresh basil leaves, for garnish
- 1 red bell pepper, roasted, peeled and seeded, quartered

DIRECTIONS:

1. Preheat oven with high heat and line a baking tray with parchment paper. Place the bell pepper on the baking tray.
2. Roast bell pepper for about 15 to 20 minutes or until the pepper starts to turn black, skin side down on the baking tray. Check the pepper regularly and remove from the oven when it starts to turn black. Set aside to cool.
3. Bring the oven temperature to 400 °F and lightly grease a muffin tin with oil.
4. Line each muffin tin with a slice of ham, making sure you don't leave spaces for the egg mix to run out.
5. Peel the skin and deseed the roasted pepper.
6. Place each slice of roasted pepper on the muffin tin together with the ham. Add 1 tablespoon of spinach on top of each pepper.
7. Top off each portion with feta cheese crumbles.
8. In a mixing bowl, combine together the egg whites,

whole egg, and then season with salt and pepper. Pour into the ham cups.

9. Bake them in the oven for about 15 minutes, or until the eggs are puffy and firm. Remove muffin tin from the oven and top off with pesto sauce, extra roasted red peppers and chopped basil. Serve.

Mediterranean Chicken Quiche

Bake this lovely quiche the night before, if you're pushed for time in the morning, and tuck a slice or two into the kids' lunchboxes for school, too.

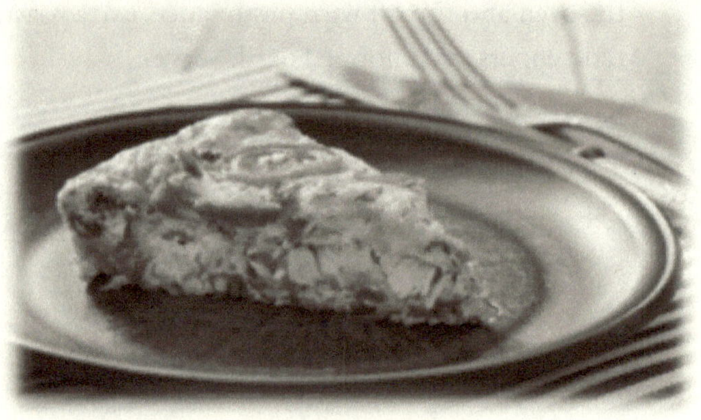

SERVES: 6

INGREDIENTS:

- ½ pound cooked chicken breast, deboned and skin removed, shredded
- 1/2 cup cherry tomatoes, halved
- 1/3 cup Feta cheese, crumbled
- 1 scallion, thinly sliced
- 2 tablespoons of fresh dill, coarsely chopped
- 2 tablespoons fresh mint leaves, coarsely chopped
- 3 large eggs
- 1 cup whole milk
- 1/4 teaspoon ground nutmeg
- Salt and freshly ground black pepper, to taste

FOR THE CRUST:

2 Med - large eggs, whisked
1/3 cup coconut oil, melted
Additional coconut oil, for greasing pie plate
3/4 cup coconut flour, sifted, preferably gluten-free

DIRECTIONS:

1. Preheat an oven to 350°F and lightly grease a 9-inch pie plate. Set aside.
2. In a medium bowl, whisk 2 eggs and oil until well incorporated. Stir in flour and blend together.
3. Add flour mix to the pie plate, press mixture with your hands until base and sides of the plate are evenly covered with crust mixture.
4. Bake it in the oven for about 10 minutes, or until light brown. Remove from the oven and set aside.
5. Increase the oven temperature to 375°F.
6. In a mixing bowl, combine together the shredded chicken, cherry tomatoes, cheese, scallions, dill and mint. Place it on top of the pie shell.
7. In separate mixing bowl, whisk together 3 eggs, milk, nutmeg, salt and pepper. Whisk it thoroughly until well incorporated, pour sauce on top of the chicken-vegetable mixture and crust.
8. Bake it in the middle rack of the oven for about 30 minutes. It is ready when a cocktail stick inserted into the thick part of quiche comes out clean, about 30 minutes. Remove from the oven and let it rest to cool before serving.

Mediterranean Beef Frittata

A frittata is an Italian version of the omelette, where instead of filling the eggs with the meats and cheese, the eggs are mixed through so that the deliciousness from the filling is all over them. You're getting in some extra veg, too, which is always a good thing!

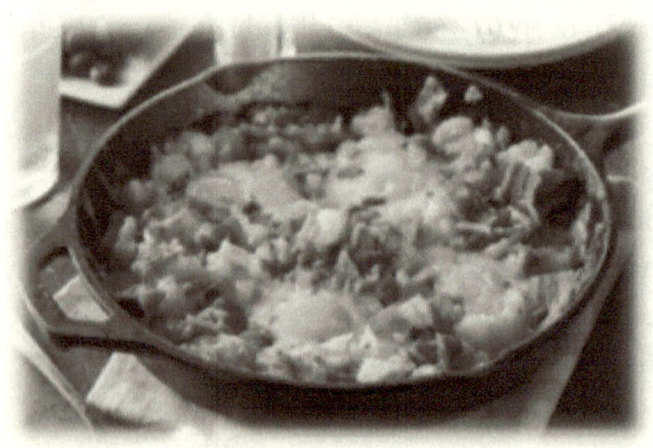

SERVES: 4

INGREDIENTS:

- 1 pound ground beef, grass-fed preferably
- 1 red bell pepper, diced
- 6 asparagus spears, chopped
- 1/2 onion, diced
- 1/2 cup canned mushrooms, quartered
- 1/2 cup arugula, chopped
- 1 tablespoon garlic, minced
- Salt and freshly ground black pepper, to taste
- 7 large eggs
- 1/4 cup milk
- 1 tablespoon of extra virgin olive oil

- 1 package of non-fat Greek yogurt (about 6 ounces)
- 1 cup Feta cheese, crumbled
- 2 tomatoes, sliced into rounds
- 1 tablespoon of dried oregano

DIRECTIONS:

1. Preheat an oven to 425°F.
2. In a pan over medium-high heat, add the oil and brown ground beef when the oil is hot, draining off any excess fat. Once beef is fully cooked and most liquid has evaporated, add the red pepper, asparagus, onions, mushrooms, arugula, garlic, season with salt and pepper. Stir to combine the ingredients evenly, cover lid and bring to a boil. Reduce to low heat and let simmer for about 10 minutes, stirring occasionally.
3. In a mixing bowl, combine together the eggs, milk, Greek yogurt and feta cheese. Whisk the ingredients thoroughly until well incorporated.
4. Lightly grease a 9-inch baking tray with oil and add in the beef and vegetable mixture. Top with egg-yogurt mixture. Give a quick stir to evenly distribute the ingredients. Garnish with sliced tomatoes and sprinkle with oregano on top.
5. Bake it in the oven for about 25 to 30 minutes, or until thoroughly cooked. It is done when a toothpick inserted in the thickest part comes out clean. Remove from oven and let it rest for about 5 to 10 minutes. Let it cool before slicing, serve with extra cheese and

Greek yogurt on top.

Mediterranean Egg Muffins

Whether you call quinoa "The Gold of the Incas" or "The Supergrain of the Future", we could all do with more of it in our diets. It is a complete protein, and contains twice the fibre of other grains, as well as good amounts of iron. In fact, this recipe is chock-full of iron because parsley and egg yolks are good sources, too.

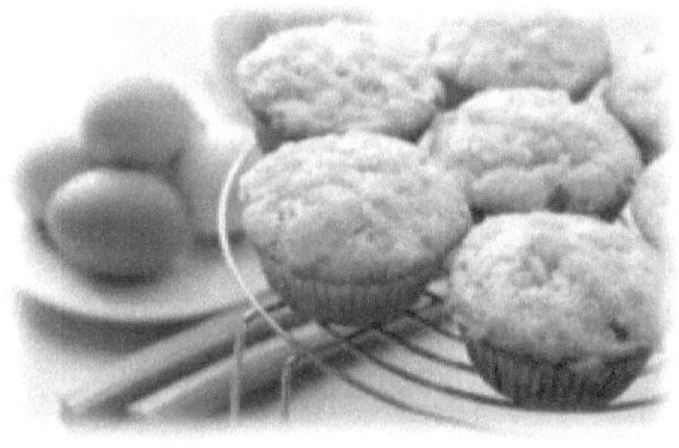

SERVES: 4

INGREDIENTS:

- 3 eggs
- 3 egg whites
- ½ cup Feta cheese, crumbled
- 1 ½ cup mixed vegetables, blanched
- 1 cup quinoa, cooked according to package directions
- 1 tablespoon onion powder
- ½ teaspoon salt, to taste
- ½ teaspoon of freshly ground black pepper, to taste
- ½ cup fresh parsley leaves, chopped
- Oil, for greasing

DIRECTIONS:

1. Preheat oven to 340°F. Lightly grease a muffin tin with oil and set aside.
2. In a mixing bowl, whisk together the eggs and egg whites for about 2 minutes or until soft peaks form.
3. Add the cheese, vegetables, quinoa, onion powder, season with salt and pepper, mix well to combine.
4. Fill each muffin tin with the mixture and bake for about 25 minutes, or until golden brown.
5. Sprinkle with chopped fresh parsley on top, let it rest to cool then serve.

Mediterranean Vegetable Cakes

Full of Mediterranean flavours such as olives, tomatoes, and artichokes, these yummy fritters are bound to become a favourite.

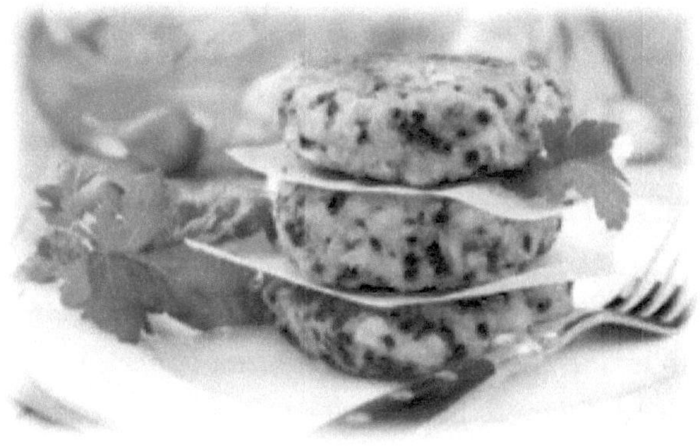

SERVES: 4

INGREDIENTS:

- 2 tablespoons of extra-virgin olive oil
- 1 medium sweet onion, diced
- 2 garlic cloves, minced
- 3 cups baby spinach,
- 1 large parsnip, peeled and grated
- 1 teaspoon of dried oregano leaves
- ¼ cup tomatoes, sun-dried, chopped
- ¼ cup Kalamata olives, chopped
- ¼ cup artichoke hearts, chopped
- 2 large eggs, lightly beaten
- ¼ cup almond flour, sifted
- ½ teaspoon of salt, to taste
- ¼ teaspoon freshly ground black pepper, to taste

DIRECTIONS:

1. Add 1 tablespoon of oil to a frying pan and place on a medium heat, once the oil is hot, add the onions and sauté until translucent and soft, stirring frequently for about 3 to 5 minutes. Add in the garlic and sauté for another minute.
2. Add the spinach, stir occasionally cooking until soft. Take off the heat and transfer it in a large bowl.
3. Stir in the grated parsnips, dried oregano, beaten eggs, sun-dried tomatoes, olives, artichokes, almond flour, and then season with black pepper and salt. Blend the ingredients well to combine. Set aside.
4. Divide the mixture into 4 equal portions.
5. In the same skillet over medium heat, add in the remaining oil. When the oil is hot, fry cakes in the skillet for 5-7 minutes on either side, or until golden and crispy. Flip it over and cook the other side for about 4 to 5 minutes.
6. Transfer it on a serving dish and serve hot. Pair with olive tapenade or mojo verde.

Mediterranean Breakfast Sandwiches

Sandwiches for breakfast? Of course, especially when they're made with toast and eggs. You won't need anything else before lunchtime after one of these.

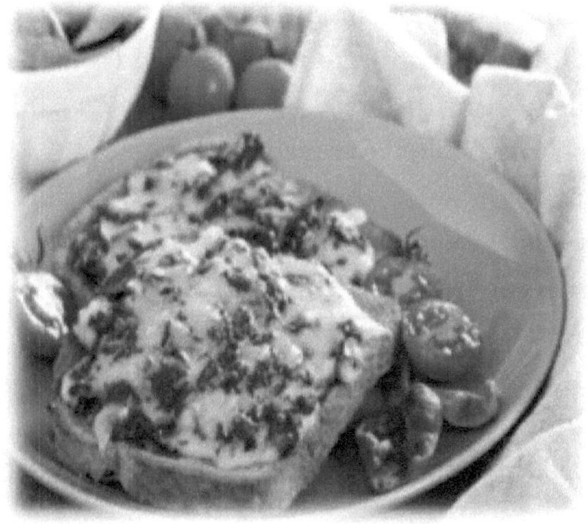

SERVES: 4

INGREDIENTS:

- 4 thin slices of multigrain sandwich
- 4 teaspoons of extra virgin olive oil
- 1 tablespoon fresh rosemary
- 4 eggs
- 2 cups fresh baby spinach leaves, blanched
- 1 medium tomato, cut into 8 thin round slices
- ¼ cup of reduced-fat Feta cheese, crumbled
- 1/8 teaspoon salt, to taste
- 1/8 teaspoon of freshly ground black pepper, to taste

DIRECTIONS:

1. Preheat oven to 375 °F.

2. Divide each sandwich into two. Set aside the half and lightly brush the other half of sandwich with olive oil. Place it on a baking sheet and toast it in the oven for about 5 minutes, or until the edges are crisp and light brown. Remove from the oven and set it aside.

3. While toasting the bread slices, heat the remaining oil in a large skillet over medium-high heat. Add the rosemary and break the eggs, cook one at a time in the skillet. Cook for about a minute or until the egg white is cooked, but the egg yolk is still runny. Remove from skillet and continue to cook the remaining eggs. Break the egg yolks, flip it over to cook the other side for another minute, or until cooked through. Remove the skillet from heat and set aside.

4. Portion the toasted sandwich on four individual serving plates. Divide the blanched baby spinach into 4 equal portions and add it on top of the sandwich. Top off each slice of sandwich with tomato slices, 1 egg, and a tablespoon of crumbled Feta cheese. Season with the salt and pepper to taste. Top with the remaining sandwich thin halves.

Potato Hash with Chickpea

You'll just have one pan to wash after making this spicy hash, flavoured with curry and ginger, and guaranteed to wake your taste buds up! Protein from the eggs and chickpeas sets you up for the day.

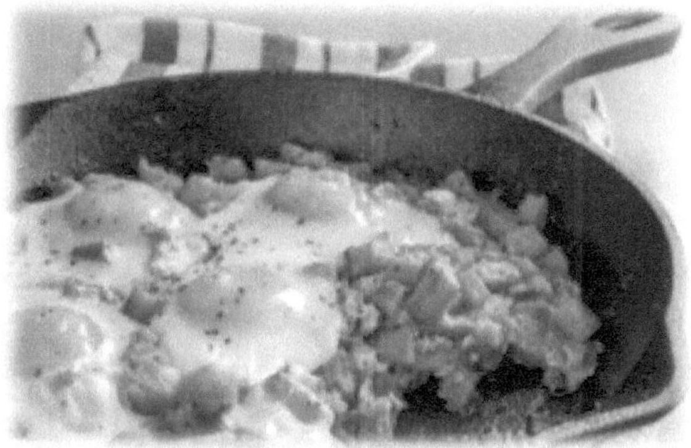

SERVES: 4 to 6

INGREDIENTS:

- 4 cups hash brown potatoes, frozen and shredded
- 2 cups baby spinach, finely chopped
- ½ cup onion, diced
- 1 tablespoon of fresh ginger root, minced
- 1 tablespoon curry powder

- salt, to taste

- ¼ cup extra-virgin olive oil
- 2 cups of canned chickpeas, rinsed and drained
- 1 large zucchini, finely chopped
- 4 large eggs

Instructions:

1. In a large bowl, combine together the shredded hash browns, chopped spinach, onion, curry powder, minced ginger, and season with salt.
2. In a non-stick skillet, heat in the oil on a medium to high heat. Drop in the potato mixture and compress into an even layer. Fry, without mixing, until the bottom is crisp and golden, this will take around 4 minutes. Once crisp turn it over and for a further 2 or 3 minutes.
3. Turn down the heat to medium-low and fold in the zucchini with the chickpeas, separating any large pieces of potato and combine the ingredients well. Press down with a wooden spoon to form a smooth layer. Make or provide 4 spaces like a well in the base for the eggs. Break the eggs, individually into a cup, carefully place it in the space provided. Continue the process with the other eggs. Place a lid over the top and cook the eggs to your preferred taste, this will take around 4 to 5 minutes.

Banana Nut Oatmeal

Quick and easy for those days when you have to rush, but don't want to compromise on good nutrition. Flaxseeds come with a host of benefits, some of them being an ability to improve blood pressure, lower fasting-glucose levels, and decrease central obesity (that "bad fat" around the waistline.) Crush them first for maximum benefit.

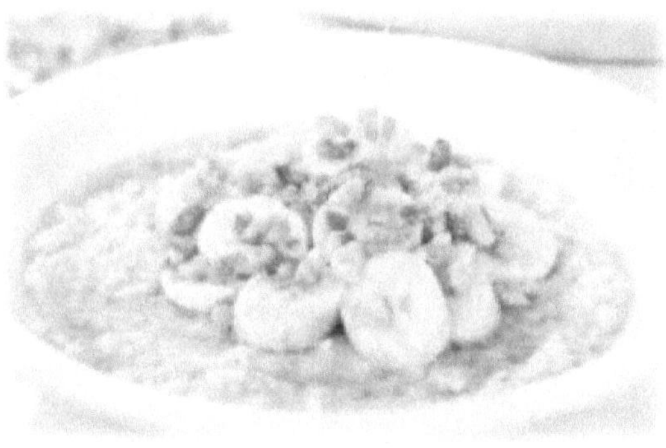

SERVES: 4

INGREDIENTS:

- ¼ cup of quick cooking oats
- ½ cup of skim milk
- 1 teaspoon flax seeds
- 2 tablespoons of walnuts, chopped
- 3 tablespoons of local honey
- 1 ripe banana, peeled and sliced into thin rounds

DIRECTIONS:

1. In a microwaveable container, combine the oats, flax seeds, banana and chopped walnuts. Stir in milk and

honey.
2. Mash the banana with a fork and add it with the mixture. Mix it thoroughly to combine the ingredients.
3. Cook in microwave on high for 2 minutes. Serve warm with whipped cream or Greek yogurt.

Melamen

Melamen is a little-known Mediterranean-style stir fry. I think of this version as an upside-down omelette!

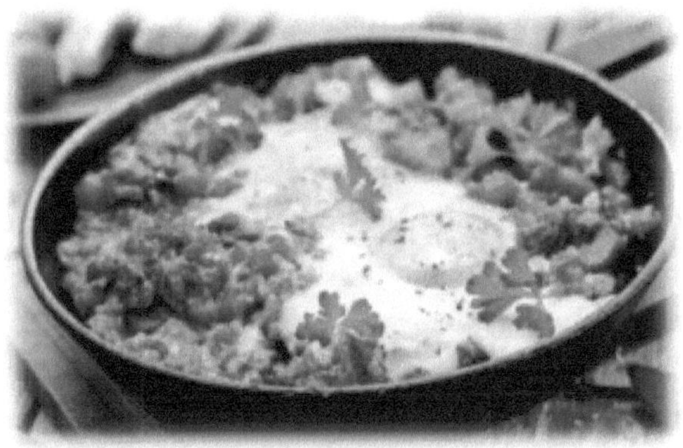

SERVES: 4

INREDIENTS:

- 1 tablespoon of extra-virgin olive oil
- 2 green bell peppers, diced
- 2 small onions, diced
- 4 medium tomatoes, diced
- 2 egg
- ½ teaspoon of salt and black pepper, to taste
- Fresh parsley leaves, for garnish

DIRECTIONS:

1. In a pan over high heat, add the olive oil and cook the green peppers for 2 minutes, covered. Reduce to medium heat and cook for another 3 minutes, or until soft.
2. While cooking the bell pepper, dice the onions and

stir them into the pan. Cover and cook again for another 1 to 2 minutes.

3. Dice the tomatoes and stir it in the pan when the onion is soft and translucent. Season with salt and pepper. Cover lid, reduce to low heat.

4. Simmer for 15 minutes with cover or until the tomatoes are soft and the melamen is still juicy. Remove pan from heat, and let the melamen rest in the pan to continue the cooking process with the heat from the pan.

5. Beat the eggs and gently pour them over the top of the melamen. Do not touch or stir the melamen, but allow the egg to be cooked on top. Serve warm.

Mediterranean Chicken Stir-Fry

This would work for dinner, too. Or lunch for that matter...Barley is good for keeping your blood sugar levels stable through the day. Studies done in Japan showed that regular barley intake significantly reduced serum cholesterol and visceral fat, both accepted markers of cardiovascular risk.

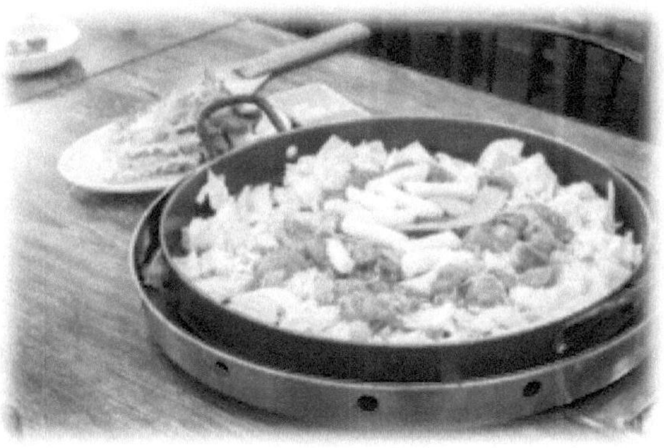

SERVES: 4

INGREDIENTS:

- 2 cups of water
- 1 cup quick-cooking barley
- 1 pound chicken breasts, deboned and skin removed, cubed
- 3 teaspoons of olive oil extra-virgin, divided
- 1 medium onion, diced
- 2 medium zucchini, cubed
- 2 garlic cloves, minced
- 1 teaspoon of dried oregano
- ½ teaspoon of dried basil leaves
- ¼ teaspoon salt, to taste
- ¼ teaspoon freshly ground black pepper, to taste

- A pinch of red pepper flakes, crushed
- 2 plum tomatoes, diced
- ½ cup pitted Greek olives, quartered
- 1 tablespoon freshly chopped parsley

DIRECTIONS:

1. In a small saucepan or pot high heat,insert the water and bring it to a boil. Stir in the barley and cover with lid. Reduce to low heat and simmer for about 10 to 12 minutes, or until barley is tender. Remove pan or pot from heat, set aside and let it stand for 5 minutes.
2. While simmering the liquid, add in 2 teaspoons of oil in a large skillet or wok. Once the oil is hot, stir-fry chicken pieces until no longer pink. Remove from wok and keep warm.
3. Stir-fry onion in remaining oil for 3 minutes. Add the zucchini, garlic, basil, oregano, seasoning and pepper flakes; stir-fry 2-4 minutes longer or until vegetables are crisp-tender. Add the chicken, olives, tomatoes, and parsley. Dish up with barley.

LEPTIN MEDITERRANEAN HEALTHY LUNCH RECIPES

While breakfast may be the most important meal of the day, lunch provides that top-up of nutrients and energy necessary to take you through the afternoon. A lunch too high in carbohydrates will cause your energy levels to plummet during the afternoon and make you sleepy, but these tasty meals will see you through the remainder of the day.

Mediterranean Salmon Salad

Try this lovely dressing with other leafy salads, too. Orzo is a quick-cooking, rice-shaped pasta, that adds a smooth texture to the salad and absorbs some of the salmon juices and delicious dressing at the same time.

SERVES: 5

INGREDIENTS:

For the Dressing

- 1/3 cup of extra-virgin olive oil
- 1/3 cup of red wine vinegar
- 1 teaspoon of dried oregano
- 1 teaspoon of onion powder
- 1/2 teaspoon of salt, to taste
- 1/2 teaspoon of freshly ground black pepper, to taste
- 1 teaspoon of Dijon mustard
- 1 teaspoon of dried basil
- 1 teaspoon of garlic powder

For the Salad

- 1 salmon filet (about ¾ pounds),
- A pinch of salt and a pinch of black pepper, to taste
- 1/4 teaspoon of dried oregano
- 1 cup dry orzo, cooked ahead according to package directions
- 1/4 cup cherry tomatoes/ olives, halved
- 1 red bell pepper, seeded and diced

- 1/2 large red onion, diced
- 1/2 cup of Feta cheese, crumbled/ Mozzarella, shredded
- 1 1/2 cups of canned artichoke hearts, drained and quartered
- 5 cups mixed leafy greens

DIRECTIONS:

1. In a mixing bowl, whisk together all ingredients except for the oil until all ingredients are well incorporated. Gradually add in small amounts of olive oil and continue to whisk until you have a thick and smooth consistency.
2. Preheat oven to 425 °F. Line a baking sheet with foil and lightly grease with oil.
3. Place salmon on a greased baking sheet lined with foil, season with salt, black pepper and oregano.
4. Bake it in the oven for about 10 to 15 minutes, or until the center is cooked through.
5. While baking the salmon, cook orzo according to package directions. Drain orzo and transfer into a casserole dish. Add in 1/4 cup of salad dressing in the casserole with the pasta, gently toss to combine. Stir in the tomatoes, feta, artichoke hearts, red bell peppers, red onions, mixed leafy greens, and the remaining salad dressing. Toss to gently combine all ingredients.
6. Once salmon is cooked, remove from the oven and flake salmon using two forks. Portion salad in

individual serving bowls/large bowl and top off with flaked salmon.

Spinach Salad with Chicken, Avocado, and Goat Cheese

A quick and substantial salad, which is also great for in a lunchbox at work or school. Just pack the dressing separately and pour over before serving.

SERVES: 4

INGREDIENTS:

FOR THE SALAD:

- 8 cups of spinach, coarsely chopped
- 1 cup of cherry tomatoes, halved
- 1/2 cup canned corn
- 1 1/2 to 2 cups of grilled/boiled chicken
- 1 large avocado, pitted and sliced
- 1/2 cup soft goat's cheese or feta cheese, crumbled
- 1/4 cup pine nuts, toasted

DRESSING:

- 2 to 3 tablespoons of white wine vinegar

- 2 tablespoons of extra-virgin olive oil
- 1 tablespoon of Dijon mustard
- salt and freshly ground black pepper, to taste

DIRECTIONS:

1. In a large salad bowl, add all salad ingredients and gently toss to combine. Stir in cooked chicken, gently toss and set aside.

2. In a separate small bowl, whisk together the entire ingredients for the dressing. Pour dressing over the salad and

gently toss. Serve with extra toasted nuts and crumbled cheese on top.

Italian Chopped Salad Recipe

Don't let the long list of ingredients put you off. Everything is quickly chopped and tossed together. Perfect when you're having friends over. Serve with a loaf of good bread for a complete meal.

SERVES: 10

INGREDIENTS:

- 3 cups of romaine lettuce, torn
- 1 cup of canned chickpeas, rinsed and drained
- 1 jar of artichoke hearts or about 6 ounces, drained and chopped
- 1 green bell pepper, diced
- 2 medium ripe tomatoes, diced
- 1/4 cup of ripe olives, drained and halved
- 1/2 cup of deli ham, diced
- 1/2 cup of hard salami, diced
- 1/2 cup pepperoni, diced
- 1/4 cup of Provolone cheese, shredded or cubed
- 2 stems of green onions, coarsely chopped
- 1/4 cup of extra-virgin olive oil
- 2 to 3 tablespoons of red wine vinegar
- 1/4 teaspoon of salt and 1/8 teaspoon of freshly ground black pepper, to taste
- 1/4 cup of shredded Parmesan cheese

DIRECTIONS:

1. In a large mixing bowl, add in romaine lettuce, chickpeas, artichoke hearts, bell pepper, tomatoes,

olives, ham, salami, pepperoni, Provolone cheese, and green onions. Set aside or chill while making the dressing.

2. To make the dressing, add and mix the oil, vinegar, salt and pepper. Whisk the ingredients until the salt is fully dissolved. Pour salad dressing over the vegetables, toss to coat. Serve with grated Parmesan cheese on top.

Greek Chicken Souvlaki Salad

Marinated then grilled chicken skewers on top of a crunchy salad, and served with a refreshing yoghurt-cucumber dip. Perfect weekend fare.

SERVES: 4

INGREDIENTS:

FOR THE CHICKEN:

- ¼ cup of extra-virgin olive oil
- 2 tablespoons of fresh lemon juice
- 2 garlic cloves, minced
- 1 teaspoon of dried oregano
- ½ teaspoon of salt, to taste
- 2 pounds of chicken breast, deboned and skin removed, cut into cubes

FOR THE SAUCE:

- ¾ cups of Greek yogurt
- ½ cucumber, peeled and seeded, grated
- 2 tablespoons of extra-virgin olive oil
- 2 to 3 tablespoons white vinegar
- 1 garlic clove, minced
- A pinch of salt

FOR THE SALAD:

- 1 medium head of Red leaf lettuce, leaves separated
- ½ cup of Feta Cheese, crumbled
- 1 cup of Pepperoncini peppers, diced and seeded
- 1 cup of Kalamata Olives

- 1 cup cherry tomatoes, halved
- ½ medium cucumber, seeded and chopped
- 1 cup canned chickpeas, rinsed and drained

DIRECTIONS:

1. Cut the chicken into bite size pieces, place it on a plate and set aside.
2. In a resealable plastic, combine together lemon juice, garlic, oil, oregano and salt. Add in the chicken, and make sure to remove air in the plastic. Refrigerate for at least two hours to marinate the meat.
3. Preheat a grill pan or charcoal grill with high heat. Soak wooden skewers in water for 30 minutes prior to cooking.
4. Place 5 to 7 pieces of marinated chicken pieces on each skewer. Cook the marinated chicken skewers in batches for 6 to 8 minutes per side, turning occasionally or until chicken is charred.
5. In a mixing bowl, add and combine the yogurt, grated cucumber, olive oil, vinegar and garlic. Season with salt and extra dried herbs to taste.
6. Portion lettuce leaves among 4 dinner plates. Top off with crumbled Feta cheese, olives, peppers, tomatoes, cucumbers and chickpeas. Place skewers on top of each plate, serve with salad dressing.

Baked Chicken Stuffed with Pesto and Cheese

Crispy chicken breast rolls with a cheesy creamy filling. Yay, I call this happy food!

SERVES: 2

INGREDIENTS:

- 2 chicken breasts, deboned and skin removed
- 2 tablespoons of lemon-basil pesto
- 2 tablespoons of sour cream, reduced fat
- 2 tablespoons of Mozzarella cheese, shredded
- 2 medium eggs, beaten
- 3 tablespoons of Parmesan cheese, finely grated
- 3 tablespoons of almond flour
- Freshly ground black pepper, as required
- Oil, for greasing

DIRECTIONS:

1. Preheat the stove to 375F. Lightly grease a small casserole using spray oil.
2. Trim excess lard from the chicken, now transfer each breast into a thick plastic bag, one at a time, pound each breast using a meat bat, so they become thin and even.
3. In a mixing bowl, combine together the sour cream, lemon-basil pesto, and shredded mozzarella cheese. Smear a layer of pesto-cream mixture with the use of a spatula covering both chicken breasts, leaving 1/2 inch clean around the chicken without the mixture. Enwrap the flattened chicken breast from the edge

with the pesto-cream mixture to the other edge. Secure each chicken roll with toothpicks.

4. Take 2 bowls for breading the chicken rolls, one bowl containing the whisked egg, in the 2nd bowl add the Parmesan and flour mixed together with salt and pepper. Dip the chicken roll in the bowl with beaten egg. Next, dredge the breast rolls in the Parmesan and flour mix, pat all sides of the breast rolls to make sure all areas are well-coated.

5. Place the chicken breasts in a greased casserole dish. Bake it in the oven for about 30 to 35 minutes, depending on the thickness of breast rolls. The breast rolls are done when it starts to turn brown to all sides. In order that the breast rolls will not be overcooked, check for doneness after 25 and 30 minutes in the oven.

6. Once the stuffed breast rolls are done, remove from the oven and let them stand for about 5 to 10 minutes. Serve whole or in round slices with leftover basil-pesto sauce.

Marsala Chicken and Mushroom Casserole

Good enough for lunch guests, but easy enough to make for the family.

SERVES: 2 to 4

INGREDIENTS:

- 2 tablespoons of unsalted butter

- 1 cup of mushrooms, halved

- 1 1/2 tablespoons of almond flour

- 1/2 cup of Marsala wine or any white wine

- 1/2 cup of heavy cream

- 2 tablespoons of fresh flat-leaf parsley, coarsely chopped

- Freshly ground black pepper and salt to taste

- 1 cup canned chickpeas, rinsed and drained

- 2 cups rotisserie chicken, cubed or cut into strips

- 2 tablespoons Parmesan cheese, grated

DIRECTIONS:

1. Preheat an oven to 350°F. Lightly grease a casserole dish with oil or butter. Set aside.

1. In a large non-stick skillet over medium –high heat, melt in the butter. Add the mushrooms and cook for

about 4 to 5 minutes, stirring occasionally until soft. Dust the cooked mushrooms with flour on top, stir and cook for another 1 minute. Stir in the wine and cream, bring to a boil and cover with lid. Reduce heat to low and simmer for about 3 minutes, stirring occasionally until smooth and thick. Stir in 2 cups of water, chopped parsley leaves, season with salt and freshly ground black pepper to taste.

1. Spread an even layer of chickpea in a greased 9-inch-by-13-inch casserole, top with the chicken pieces. Pour over the mushroom gravy on top, Cover tightly with a foil and bake for about 35 minutes or until visible bubbles moves to the top surface. Remove and discard the foil, sprinkle with grated parmesan cheese on top. Return casserole in the oven, bake for 5 minutes in order to brown and melt the cheese. Remove from the oven and let it stand for about 5 to 10 minutes before serving.

Low-Carb Tuscan Soup

Rich and aromatic, this soup will easily serve a crowd.

SERVES: 14

INGREDIENTS:

- 2 tablespoons of unsalted butter
- 2 cups of Turkey Italian Sausage, casing removed and sliced into thin rounds
- 6 cups of low-sodium beef broth
- 2 cups of kale, chopped
- 1 head of cauliflower, detached florets
- 6 cloves of garlic, minced
- 3 medium slices of bacon, sliced into small pieces
- 1 cup of heavy whipping cream

DIRECTIONS:

1. In a deep stock pot over medium-high heat, melt in the butter and brown sausage for about 5 to 7 minutes. Remove sausage from the pot then add the bacon and onion in the same pot. Cook until the onion is soft and translucent, about 10 minutes and add the garlic. Cook for another 3 to 4 minutes, or until the garlic brown and aromatic.
2. Add 6 cups of beef broth and vegetables. Bring it to a steady boil for 35 minutes with lid on.
3. Remove pot from heat and stir in the heavy cream before serving. Add the sausage on top.

Crockpot Low -Carb Spicy Chicken Soup

Creamy and convenient, if you put this in the crockpot quickly after breakfast, it will be ready in time for lunch.

SERVES: 8

INGREDIENTS:

- 4 cups water
- 3 chicken breasts. Shredded
- 1/2 large onion, diced
- 1/4 head of cabbage, in chiffonades
- 1 cup tinned stewed tomatoes
- 1 /2 cup of tinned red chillies
- 1 cup of salsa
- 1 cup cream cheese, softened
- 4 tablespoons heavy whipping cream
- 1 tablespoon garlic salt
- 1 tablespoon ground cumin
- Salt and black pepper, to taste

DIRECTIONS:

1. In the crock pot with 4 cups of water, place chicken breasts, onion and cabbage.
2. Cook for about 4 hours with high heat, or 6 to 8 hours on low until chicken is done. Take chicken out of the broth, cool and shred the meat into bite size pieces.
3. Return the chicken back in the pot, add the remaining ingredients and cook until cream cheese has melted and soup is thick and creamy.

4. Serve with sour cream on the side.

Low-Carb Avgolemono (Greek Chicken, Lemon & Egg Soup)

Fresh- tasting and light, this soup is also quick to make.

SERVES: 8

INGREDIENTS:

- 4 cups cooked, shredded chicken
- 10 cups chicken broth or stock
- 3 eggs
- 1/3 cup fresh lemon juice
- 2 cups cooked spaghetti squash
- 1/4 cup fresh parsley
- salt and pepper to taste
- 1 lemon, sliced into wedges
- freshly grated parmesan cheese (optional)

DIRECTIONS:

1. In a pot over high heat, add the broth and chicken breast. Bring it to a steady boil for 5 minutes, remove pot from heat.
2. In a mixing bowl, whisk the eggs and lemon juice until thick and frothy.
3. Gradually add in small amounts of 2 cups stock into the egg mixture, stirring constantly. Add the hot stock slowly and in gradual amounts to avoid cooking the eggs.
4. Once the chicken stock and the egg mixture are well incorporated, return the mixture in the pot.
5. Add in the spaghetti squash and season with salt and

pepper to taste. Reheat the soup with low heat if needed and avoid the soup from boiling.

6. Serve warm with lemon wedges and fresh herbs on top.

Cream of Roasted Cauliflower Soup, with Cumin, Paprika, and Fresh Dill

This is a creamy, satisfying soup, with the flavours of hummus. If you don't have sumac, substitute some lemon zest instead.

SERVES: 5 to 6

INGREDIENTS:

- 2 medium heads of detached cauliflower florets
- 3 tablespoons of olive oil
- olive oil, for greasing
- Kosher salt, to taste
- Black pepper, to taste
- 1 small onion, diced
- 2 tablespoons of minced garlic
- ¼ to ½ of turmeric powder
- 1 to 2 teaspoons of sumac powder
- ½ tablespoon of cumin powder
- 2 ½ teaspoons Spanish paprika
- 4 to 5 cups of organic vegetable stock
- 1 cup water
- 2 to 2 ½ cups heavy cream
- 1 organic lemon, freshly juiced
- 1 cup fresh dill, coarsely chopped

DIRECTIONS:

1. Preheat the oven with a temperature of 425 °F. Lightly grease a baking sheet with oil, set aside.
2. Place the detached florets of cauliflower on the

bottom of the greased baking sheet. Lightly brush with olive oil and dust with pepper and salt over the top.

3. Roast the vegetables for about 25 to 30 minutes, flipping over to cook the other side after the first 15 minutes. Remove vegetables from oven and let it rest

4. Meanwhile, heat 2 tablespoons olive oil in a large heavy pot or Dutch oven. In the heated oil, sauté onion until translucent. Add chopped garlic, cumin, turmeric, paprika and sumac. Stir together for a brief few seconds until fragrant.

5. Next add in ¾ of the roasted cauliflower, keep the rest for later. Stir to coat cauliflower well with the spices then add vegetable broth and water.

6. Bring to a simmer on medium-high heat. Cover and cook for five minutes or until cauliflower is aldenté as it takes in the liquid.

7. Uncover and remove from heat momentarily. Using and immersion blender, blend the cauliflower with the liquid until you reach a desired smoothness.

8. Return to a medium heat and stir in heavy cream with the lemon juice. Then add in the rest of roasted cauliflower florets you reserved earlier. Cook for a few minutes to warm the soup through. Test and add a pinch of salt if needed.

9. Finally, stir in the chopped dill.

10. Serve hot with your favorite bread.

LEPTIN MEDITERRANEAN HEALTHY DINNER RECIPES

In keeping with the leptin-friendly principle of having a light evening meal, and having it early, we've designed these recipes to be quick to make, and never heavy or too rich. We have some lovely seafood options, as well as vegetarian recipes for those meat-free Mondays, and also a beefy salad for when you crave a little red meat with your dinner.

Mediterranean Shrimp over Spinach

This is a quick weekday dinner, but much better than ordinary "fast food." Just be careful not to overcook the shrimp.

SERVES: 4

INGREDIENTS:

- 2 cups tinned diced tomatoes, drained
- 2 tablespoons of capers
- 2 cups of spinach leaves
- 1/2 large onion, diced
- 1 teaspoon garlic, finely minced
- 2 tablespoons olive oil, divided
- 1 large green bell pepper, deseeded and diced
- 1 teaspoon of Italian Herb Blend
- 1/2 cup fish stock
- salt and freshly ground black pepper, to taste
- 1 pound fresh large shrimp, shelled and deveined

DIRECTIONS:

1. In a large pan over medium-high heat, add 1 tablespoon of olive oil. Once the oil is hot, sauté the onion and green bell pepper for about 3 to 4 minutes. Stir in the minced garlic and Italian herb, and then cook for another 2 minutes, stirring occasionally.
2. Add the diced tomatoes and fish stock, cover lid and bring to a boil. Reduce to low heat and simmer for 10 minutes.
3. In a separate pan, apply medium-high heat and add the oil. Once the oil is hot, add the spinach and cook

for about 2 to 3 minutes, stirring occasionally. Remove pan from heat, set aside.

4. In the pan with sautéed vegetables, add the shrimp and capers. Cook for about 4 to 5 minutes or until the shrimp turns opaque in color. Season with salt and pepper to taste, cook for another minute.

5. Portion spinach into serving bowls and top with shrimp and capers. Serve hot.

Mediterranean Low-Carb "Cauliflower Risotto"

This is more foolproof than a traditional risotto, and eliminates the risk of gluey rice.

SERVES: 4

INGREDIENTS:

- 1 medium head cauliflower , detaches florets
- 2 tablespoons freshly chopped basil-oregano-thyme
- 2 tablespoons clarified butter
- ½ cup pesto sauce
- 2 cloves garlic, mashed
- 4 medium chicken breasts, skinned and deboned, diced
- ¼ cup heavy whipping cream or coconut milk
- ½ organic lemon, zested
- Pinch of freshly ground black pepper
- ½ teaspoon pink Himalayan[1] or sea salt[2], to taste
- 1 cup Parmesan cheese, grated

DIRECTIONS:

1. Put the cauliflower florets in blender, pulse until you have a coarse texture to imitate the rice.
2. In a pan over medium-high heat, melt in the butter and add the diced chicken. Cook chicken for about 15 minutes, remove from pan. Transfer on a dish, set aside.
3. In the same pan over medium heat, melt in the

---

1. http://amzn.to/1sUj6ox

2. http://amzn.to/1jIIwWe

remaining butter and cook lemon zest and garlic for about 3 to 4 minutes or until golden.

4. Add the cauliflower rice in the pan and cook for another 5 minutes, stirring constantly. Add the pesto sauce, cream and chopped herbs. Cook for another 2 to 3 minutes. Season to taste with salt and pepper.

5. Portion into serving plates, top off with grated Parmesan cheese. Serve warm.

Mediterranean Baked Fish, with Tomato- Onion- Garlic Sauce

Try this with any white fish. The delicious sauce keeps the fish from drying out in the oven.

SERVES: 4

INGREDIENTS:

- 1 teaspoon ground fennel seeds
- 1/2 teaspoon dried oregano
- 1 bay leaf
- 1 garlic clove, minced
- 3/4 cup of apple juice
- 1/2 cup tomato juice
- 1 1/2 teaspoon of dried thyme, crushed
- 1/2 teaspoon of dried basil, crushed
- 2 teaspoons olive oil extra virgin
- 1 Med - large onion, diced
- 2 cups canned whole tomatoes, drained and diced
- 4 cups of lemon juice
- 1/4 cup of orange juice
- 1 tablespoon freshly grated orange peel
- black pepper, to taste
- 1 pound flounder fillets

DIRECTIONS:

1. In a skillet, apply medium heat and add the oil. Once the oil is hot, sauté the onions for about 4 minutes or until soft and translucent.
2. Stir in all of the remaining ingredients except for the

fish. Stir it thoroughly, cover with a lid and simmer for about 30 minutes.

3. Preheat an oven to 350°F.

4. Grease a baking dish and add the fish fillets. Pour over the sauce to cover.

5. Bake in the oven for about 15 minutes or until the fish easily flakes.

Shrimp Saganaki

Saganaki is a Greek appetizer, made with a thick slice of cheese, dusted with flour and then fried till the middle is melted. It gets its name from the small two-handled heavy frying pan in which it's made. It's basically a chunk of fried cheese for a meze platter, but in this version it's made into a complete meal with the addition of shrimp and some vegetables.

SERVES: 4

INGREDIENTS:

- 12 large shrimp, deveined and peeled
- 1/2 cup Chardonnay wine
- 1/2 cup Feta cheese, crumbled
- 1 tablespoon of extra-virgin olive oil
- 1 medium fennel bulb, cored and finely diced
- 2 tablespoons lemon juice, divided
- 1/4 teaspoon salt
- 5 scallions, finely cut
- 1 chilli pepper, such as jalapeño or Serrano, seeded and minced
- Ground black pepper, to taste

DIRECTIONS:

1. In a bowl, add shrimp, salt and lemon juice. Toss and set aside.
2. In a skillet, apply medium heat and add the oil. Once the oil is hot, add scallions, fennel and chilli pepper. Cook for about 4 to 5 minutes, stirring constantly until soft. Add in the wine, cook for another minute and add the shrimp on top of the sautéed ingredients. Cook with lid on, for about 4 minutes. Remove skillet from heat.
3. Transfer the shrimp on a serving dish. Add the remaining lemon juice, pepper and Feta in the skillet and cook until the cheese is melted.
4. Transfer the vegetables on a serving dish and top off with shrimp. Serve warm.

Grilled Shrimp Salad with Feta, Tomato, and Watermelon
This pretty salad combines all the colors of the Italian flag, and then gets topped with delicious flame-grilled shrimp skewers.

SERVES: 4
INGREDIENTS:

- 1/4 cup extra-virgin olive oil
- 1-1/2 teaspoon of local honey
- Vegetable oil, for the grill
- 1 1/2 pound large fresh shrimp, peeled and deveined
- 1/4 cup and 2 tablespoon fresh lemon juice
- 1 teaspoon paprika
- salt and freshly cracked black pepper, to taste
- 1/2 medium head of frisée, torn into small pieces
- 3 cups watermelon, deseeded and diced
- 3 red tomatoes, cut into wedges
- 2 cups cherry tomatoes, cut into halves
- ¾ cup Feta cheese, diced
- 1/2 cup fresh basil leaves, shredded

DIRECTIONS:

1. Prepare a gas or charcoal grill, and preheat with high heat.
2. Mix lemon juice and paprika in a mixing bowl, stir in the shrimp. Toss to coat, set aside and marinate for about 5 minutes. Season shrimp with salt and pepper, thread into skewers.
3. Mix together ¼ cup lemon juice, honey, oil, and a

pinch of pepper and salt. Mix it thoroughly, set aside.

4. Scrape off the burnt food in the cooking grates and brush with oil. Grill the skewered shrimps, flipping occasionally to cook them evenly. Cook for about 5 to 6 minutes in total, or until opaque and firm.

5. In a mixing bowl, toss in the tomatoes, basil, cheese, watermelon, 2 tablespoon of dressing, salt and pepper. In a separate mixing bowl, toss frisée with 3 tablespoons of dressing and portion into serving bowls. Portion into each serving bowl the watermelon-tomato mixture and top off with shrimp skewers. Drizzle with the remaining dressing on top, serve.

Orecchiette with Mussels & Mint

This dish packs big flavour with just a few ingredients. It's quick to make, too.

SERVES: 4

INGREDIENTS:

- 1 tablespoon of salt
- 2 medium zucchini, cut into batonnets
- 1/2 cup heavy cream
- 1 recipe of orecchiette[3]
- A dozen of mussels, cleaned
- 1/2 cup dry white wine
- Salt and freshly ground black pepper, to taste
- 1/4 cup fresh mint leaves, chopped

DIRECTIONS:

1. Add water in a pot over high heat, bring to a boil and add salt and orecchiette. Cook for about 8 minutes or until done.
2. In a frying pan, add the mussels and wine, apply medium heat and cover. Bring to a boil and cook for about 2 to 3 minutes, or until the mussels have opened. Remove the mussels with a slotted spoon, strain the mussel stock with cheesecloth and return in the pan. Add the zucchini, return to a boil and simmer for about 3 minutes or until soft.
3. Remove the shells of the mussels, discard shells and add the meat in the pan with the zucchini.

---

3. http://www.finecooking.com/recipes/basic-orecchiette-pasta.aspx

Stir in the cream, season with salt and pepper.

1. Toss the orecchiette into the pan, cook until the sauce starts to thicken, or for about 2 minutes. Top off with mint, serve.

Greek-Style Shrimp Salad

A lovely light dinner dish, where the tang of olives and capers
are balanced with the creaminess of the cheese.

SERVES: 4

INGREDIENTS:

- 1 pound of fresh, large shrimps, peeled and deveined
- 1/4 cup pitted black olives, chopped
- 1 tablespoon capers, drained and rinsed
- 5 tablespoons of extra-virgin olive oil
- 1 teaspoon dried oregano
- salt and coarsely ground black pepper, to taste
- 1 cup plum tomatoes, diced and seeded
- ½ cup Feta cheese or goat's cheese, crumbled
- 1 tablespoon red wine vinegar
- 1 tablespoon fresh lemon juice, organic
- 1 cup baby greens, washed and drained

DIRECTIONS:

1. Preheat a broiler to high and place an oven rack on
   top rung.
2. Mix together the oil, salt and pepper in a bowl and
   toss in the shrimp. Cover a baking sheet with foil and
   layer the shrimp on it. Broil the shrimp for about 5
   minutes, or until opaque inside and pink on the
   outside.
3. While broiling the shrimp, combine capers, lemon
   juice, feta, olives, tomatoes, oregano, oil, vinegar and
   the remaining lemon juice in a mixing bowl. When

the shrimp is done, toss it with tomato-feta mixture.

4. Add the greens, toss to combine and portion into individual serving bowls. Serve with extra herbs and cheese on top.

Halibut and Mussel Stew with Fennel, Peppers, and Saffron

Use the crunchy garlic toasts to mop up all the delicious juices.

SERVES: 4

INGREDIENTS:

- 2 tablespoons olive oil, extra-virgin
- 1 yellow onion, sliced thinly
- 1 fennel bulb, trimmed and quartered
- salt and freshly ground black pepper, to taste
- 4 baguette slices, 1 inch thick
- 2 to 3 tablespoons of tomato paste
- 2 cloves of garlic, crushed
- 1/2 cup dry white wine (Albariño)
- 1 carrot, peeled and sliced thinly
- 1 ½ cup of halibut fillets, cut into bite size pieces
- 1 dozen of fresh mussels, cleaned
- 2 pinches of saffron
- 1 bay leaf
- 1 red bell pepper, seeded and sliced into strips
- 1 cup canned chickpeas, drained and rinsed
- 1 teaspoon fresh thyme leaves, minced
- A pinch of pimenton

DIRECTIONS:

1. In a saucepan with oil over medium heat, add the onion, fennel, carrot, and bell pepper. Cook for about 5 to 6 minutes, stirring it until the vegetables

are tender.

2. Stir in the tomato paste and garlic in the saucepan, cook for about 1 minute. Stir constantly and add in the wine. Cover lid and bring to a simmer, cook until thickened and reduced by half. Add 3 cups of water, chickpeas, bay leaf, thyme, pimenton and saffron. Bring to a boil and cover, cook for about 20 to 25 minutes or vegetables are tender and sauce has thickened. Season with salt and black pepper to taste.

3. Preheat the broiler on high, place the bread slices brushed with oil on a baking sheet. Broil for about 2 minutes on each side, flipping once to cook the other side until golden-brown.

4. Remove bread from the oven and rub with crushed garlic, place it on a serving dish.

5. Add the halibut and mussels into the pan with the stew, cover and simmer for about 4 to 8 minutes, or until the fish is cooked and all the mussels have opened.

6. Ladle stew into shallow bowls, serve with the garlic toasts.

Tilapia Feta Florentine

A richly satisfying bake, full of nutritious goodness.

SERVES: 4

INGREDIENTS:

- 1 garlic clove, minced
- 2 cups of fresh spinach, chopped
- 1/4 cup olives, sliced
- 1 tablespoon of olive oil
- 1/4 cup onion, diced
- ½ teaspoon of dried oregano
- ½ teaspoon of white pepper
- 2 tablespoons Feta cheese or goat's cheese, crumbled
- 1/2 teaspoon zest lemon rind
- 1/2 teaspoon salt, to taste
- 3 to 4 tilapia fillets
- 2 tablespoons of unsalted butter, melted
- 2 teaspoons of fresh lemon juice
- 1 pinch paprika, to taste

DIRECTIONS:

1. Preheat an oven to 400°F. Grease a 9x13 baking dish, set aside.
2. In a skillet over medium-high heat, heat the oil. Once the oil is hot, sauté the garlic and onion for about 4 minutes, or until soft and fragrant. Stir in the spinach and cook for 4 minutes until wilted. Add in the lemon zest, oregano, pepper, olives, cheese and salt to the skillet. Cook for another 4 minutes or until the

cheese has melted.

3. Lay the spinach on the greased baking dish and place tilapia on top. Drizzle with butter-lemon mixture and sprinkle with smoked paprika.

4. Bake it in oven for 20 to 25 minutes, or until the fish is flaky and cooked through.

1.

Gyro Salad

A delicious green salad topped with strips of seasoned beef

SERVES: 4

INGREDIENTS:

YOGURT DRESSING:

- ½ cup Greek yogurt
- ½ cup reduced-fat sour cream
- ¼ cup milk
- 1 teaspoon of Greek seasoning

SALAD:

- 1 sirloin steak beef or about 1 pound, cut into strips
- 1 tablespoon of extra virgin olive oil
- 2 teaspoons of Greek seasoning
- 8 cups of mixed salad greens
- 1 medium cucumber, seeded and thinly sliced
- 1 red onion, sliced into thin rounds
- 1 large ripe tomato, diced

DIRECTIONS:

1. In a mixing bowl, whisk together all of the dressing ingredients until smooth and creamy.
2. In a skillet over medium-high heat, add the oil. Once the oil is hot, add the beef and the Greek seasoning. Cook until beef is brown, stirring frequently for about 5 to 7 minutes. Drain if necessary.
3. Portion salad greens on serving plates and top off

with cucumber, onion, tomato and strips of beef.
Serve with dressing on top.

LEPTIN MEDITERRANEAN HEALTHY SOUP RECIPES

Soup is a great option for a light dinner, or for those times when you're feeling peckish but want a healthy snack. It's the ultimate fast food too, as many soups can be cooked within half an hour. Preparation is usually done in one pot, leaving you with less washing up to do!

Many of the soups in this chapter will freeze well, so you could make a batch and freeze single portions for convenience.

Cabbage Soup with Kielbasa

Kielbasa is a type of smoked sausage, which pairs perfectly with cabbage in this soup which is bursting both with flavour and goodness.

SERVES: 4

INGREDIENTS:

- 2 cups of Kielbasa, sliced into thin rounds
- 2 cups of cabbage, cut into chiffonades
- 2 medium zucchini, sliced into rounds
- 2 green pepper, diced
- 2 tablespoon extra-virgin olive oil
- 2 small yellow pepper, diced
- 1 medium onion, diced
- 2 cups of tomato juice
- 1 cup of canned stewed tomatoes
- 2 cups vegetable stock
- 1 tablespoon red hot chilli powder
- ½ teaspoon of ground black pepper
- ½ teaspoon salt
- 1 medium stalk celery , chopped
- ½ cup of fresh mushrooms, quartered

DIRECTIONS:

1. In a pan, apply medium-high heat and add 1 tablespoon of oil. Once the oil is hot, add the onion, diced peppers, and celery. Cook for about 5 minutes until soft and tender. Stir in the mushrooms and cook for another 3 minutes. Remove pan from heat, set

aside.

2. In a separate pan, apply medium-high heat and add the oil. Add in sliced Kielbasa and cook for about 4 to 5 minutes. Stir in the sautéed vegetables and cook for 2 to 3 minutes, stirring occasionally. Add in the stewed tomatoes, tomato juice, chilli powder and season with the seasoning. Heat to a boil, then turn the heat to low and simmer for 5 minutes, stirring occasionally. Remove from heat, set aside.

3. In a large saucepan, pour in the vegetable stock and heat to a boil. Blanche the zucchini in the boiling stock for about 2 to 3 minutes, remove from pot and transfer into a bowl with ice bath. Drain zucchini and set aside. Blanche the cabbage for about 2 minutes in the pot, remove from pot and place into a bowl with ice bath. Drain and set aside.

4. In the pot, stir in the simmered ingredients from the pan and bring to a boil. Add the blanched vegetables and return to a boil. Remove pot from heat, portion soup into serving bowls. Serve warm.

Chilled Red Pepper Soup with Sautéed Shrimp

Serve this refreshing soup in the summer months, when a hot dinner is just not what you feel like.

SERVES: 6

INGREDIENTS:

- 1 cup croutons
- 2 garlic cloves, mashed into paste
- 1 cucumber, peeled and deseeded, chopped
- 1 lemon, sliced into wedges
- ½ cup canned/jarred roasted red peppers, diced
- 2 cups tomato juice
- 1/2 teaspoon ground cumin
- 4 tablespoons extra-virgin olive oil
- 3 tablespoons cider vinegar
- Salt and coarsely ground black pepper
- 2 dozen small shrimps, peeled and deveined
- 1 tablespoon fresh thyme leaves, minced
- ½ cup fish stock

DIRECTIONS:

1. In a food processor or blender, add the cucumber, red pepper, tomato juice, croutons, 4 tablespoons of oil and 2 tablespoons of vinegar. Add ½ cup fish stock and pulse until smooth, season with cumin, salt and pepper and pulse again until you have a thick and smooth mixture. Transfer into a bowl, cover and chill in the fridge.
2. In a pan, apply medium-high heat and add the

remaining oil. Once the oil is hot, add the garlic paste and shrimp. Cook for 5 minutes, stirring occasionally. Season with salt and pepper to taste. Cool and chill in the refrigerator.

3. Remove the chilled soup and portion into individual serving bowls. Top off with minced thyme and peeled shrimp, and serve with lemon wedges.

Grilled Watermelon Gazpacho with Lime Cream

A very refreshing chilled soup, perfect for a summer evening.

SERVES: 5

INGREDIENTS:

- 2 medium tomatoes, diced
- 2 medium cucumber, peeled and cubed
- 2 tablespoons extra-virgin olive oil
- 1 Serrano chilli, deseeded and diced
- 1 organic lime, juiced
- 1 teaspoons chipotle chilli powder
- 1 medium watermelon , sliced into wedges
- Kosher salt, to taste
- 1/4 cup fresh cilantro, minced
- 1 shallot, minced
- 1 to 2 tablespoons red wine vinegar
- 1/4 cup crème fraîche

DIRECTIONS:

1. Prepare a charcoal or gas grill set up, preheat to high.
2. In a small bowl, combine 1 tablespoon of oil, salt and chipotle. Lightly brush the watermelon with the mixture. Grill for about 2 minutes on each side, or until nicely charred. Remove from grill and set aside to cool. Remove the rinds and seeds, and dice the flesh.
3. In a food processor, add the watermelon, tomato, cilantro, shallot, cucumber, chilli and the remaining

oil. Pulse for 1 minute and add half of the lime juice and vinegar. Pulse again until you have a smooth and thick mixture. Season with salt and pepper, place in a bowl and chill for at least 2 hours.

4. Before serving, combine crème fraîche and the remaining lime juice in a bowl. Portion soup into individual serving bowls, drizzle with cream-lime mixture on top.

White Gazpacho with Grapes and Toasted Almonds
Gazpacho is a cold soup, with Spanish origins.
SERVES: 4
INGREDIENTS:

- 3 slices of white bread, edges trimmed, soaked
- ¼ cup almonds
- 2 medium cucumbers, deseeded and diced
- 1/2 cup of warm water
- 3 cloves garlic, peeled and crushed
- 1 tablespoon of fresh organic lemon juice, or as needed to taste
- 5 scallions, green parts trimmed off and thinly sliced
- 1/4 cup sherry vinegar, or as needed to taste
- 1/2 teaspoon of salt, or as needed to taste
- 3 tablespoons of extra-virgin olive oil
- ½ cup green grapes, halved

DIRECTIONS:

1. In a pan, apply medium-high heat and toast the almonds in. Cook for 4 to 5 minutes until browned and fragrant, tossing occasionally. Remove from pan, set aside.

2. Reserve ¼ of cucumber, 1 tablespoon almonds, and 1 tablespoon of scallion for garnish, set aside. In a food processor, add the remaining cucumber, crushed garlic, soaked bread, scallions, vinegar, lemon juice, almonds, salt and oil. Pulse until you have a uniform-sized mixture of ingredients and add more salt and

vinegar, if needed. Pulse again until a smooth and thick mixture is achieved.

3. Portion into individual serving bowls, serve with cucumber, scallions, grapes and toasted almonds on top.

Mediterranean Kale & White Bean Soup with Sausage
SERVES: 6 to 8
INGREDIENTS:

- 3 links of sweet Italian sausage, casings removed and chopped
- Salt and coarsely ground black pepper
- 5 cups chicken broth
- 1 carrot, peeled and diced
- 1 celery stalk, cut into small dice
- ½ pound kale, stems removed and leaves coarsely chopped
- 2 tablespoons of fresh organic lemon juice
- 2 tablespoons of olive oil
- Pinch of red pepper flakes, crushed
- 2 cups of cooked dried beans
- 1 small yellow onion, diced
- 4 garlic cloves, minced
- 1/2 teaspoon zest of lemon

DIRECTIONS:

1. Heat 1 tablespoon of oil in a large saucepan and place on a medium-high heat. Put in the sausage and fry for about 4 minutes, occasionally stir. Remove from pot, transfer into a plate and leave the oil.
2. Add the remaining oil in the pot. Add the onion and cook for about 2 minutes, stirring occasionally. Stir in the carrot and celery, cook for another 2 minutes until browned and tender. Stir in the garlic, pepper

flakes, ground black pepper and salt in the pot. Cook
for 2 minutes until the garlic is fragrant, add the
broth and reduce heat to high.

3. Add the sausage and half of the beans, mash
    remaining beans and add into the pot. Cover lid and
    bring to a boil. When it starts to boil, add the kale
    and reduce heat to low and simmer for 15 minutes.
    Add the lemon zest and juice, adjust seasoning to
    desired taste.

4. Remove pot from heat and portion soup into
    individual serving bowls. Serve warm.

Moroccan Vegetable Ragoût

A ragoût is a traditional French stew, and the name literally means "to revive the taste." This lovely vegetarian option will certainly revive your taste buds, as well as deliver a good dose of vitamins at the same time.

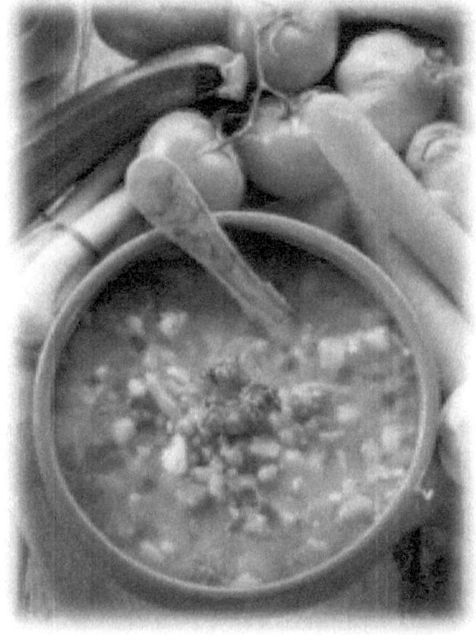

SERVES: 3 to 4

INGREDIENTS:

- 1 tablespoon olive oil, extra-virgin
- 1 orange, juiced
- 2 teaspoons of local honey
- 1 yellow onion, thinly sliced
- 2 cups sweet potatoes, peeled and diced
- 2 cups canned chickpeas, drained and rinsed
- 1 cup canned diced tomatoes
- 1 cinnamon stick
- 1 cup vegetable stock

- 2 teaspoons ground cumin
- ½ cup green Greek or Italian olives, pitted
- 2 cups kale leaves, lightly packed and chopped
- Kosher salt and roughly ground black pepper, to taste

DIRECTIONS:

1. In a pot over medium-high heat, add the oil. When hot, put in the onion and cook for about 4 minutes until soft and translucent. Add cinnamon stick, cumin, potatoes, tomatoes, chickpeas, olives, orange juice, honey and stock in the pot. Cover lid and bring to a boil.

2. Once it starts to boil, reduce to low heat and simmer for 15 minutes. Add in the kale and give it a quick stir and cover. Simmer for another 10 minutes, or Up to the vegetables are soft and tender. Season with salt and black pepper to taste.

3. Remove pot from heat, portion soup into serving bowls and serve warm.

Cucumber-Yogurt Soup with Avocado

Another chilled soup: pretty, light, and packed full of vitamins.

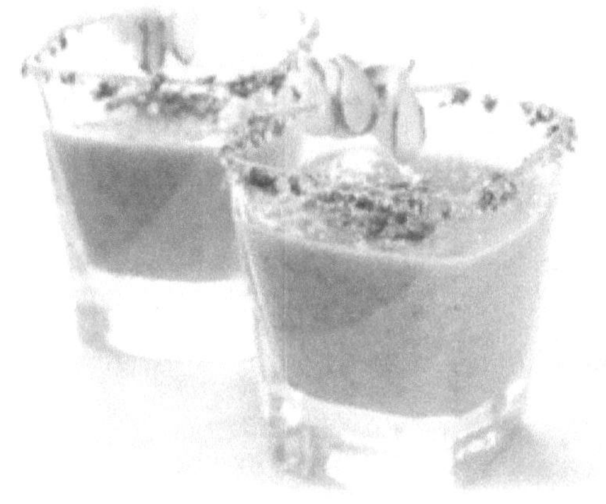

SERVES: 4
INGREDIENTS:

- 2 tablespoons extra-virgin olive oil
- 1 teaspoon garlic, minced
- 2 medium cucumbers, peeled and seeded, diced
- 1 medium ripe avocado, peeled and pitted, diced
- 1 cup plain yogurt
- 1 teaspoon toasted cumin seeds, ground
- 1 teaspoon salt, or as needed to taste
- 1 large white onion, diced
- 2 tablespoons minced fresh basil leaves
- 2 tablespoons minced fresh mint leaves
- 3 tablespoons fresh lemon juice
- Coarsely ground black pepper, as needed to taste

•

DIRECTIONS:

1. Add the onion and cucumber in a food processor, pulse until a coarse mixture is achieved. Take out ½ cup of the onion-cucumber mixture, place it in a bowl and set aside.
2. Add the avocado in the processor, together with oil, yogurt, garlic and season with cumin and salt. Purée the ingredients until a smooth consistency is achieved.
3. Place the puréed ingredients in a bowl, stir in the basil, mint, lemon juice, remaining onion-cucumber mixture and ½ cup of water. Stir to combine, adjust consistency by adding more water and then season with salt and pepper. Cover and chill for at least 1 hour before serving.
4. Portion chilled soup into individual serving bowls. Serve.

Roasted Red Pepper & Tomato Gazpacho

While the cheese at the end is optional, it does add a lovely ontrast in texture, flavour, and color.

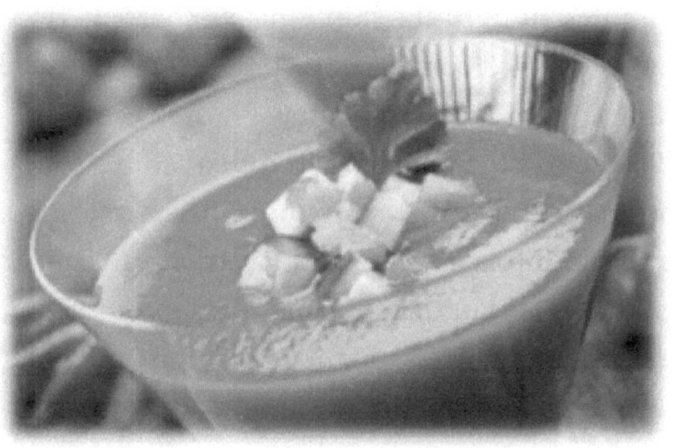

SERVES: 4

INGREDIENTS:

- 2 red bell peppers, seeded and halved
- 3 cups of ripe tomatoes, seeded and diced
- 3 garlic cloves, minced
- 4 tablespoons extra-virgin olive oil, or as needed
- 1 organic lemon, juiced
- 4 scallions, chopped
- 2 cucumbers, peeled and seeded, diced
- 1/2 cup mixed fresh herbs, chopped (thyme, chervil, basil, parsley, marjoram, and tarragon)
- salt and coarsely ground black pepper, to taste
- 1/4 cup goat's cheese, crumbled (optional)

DIRECTIONS:

1. Roast the peppers in a preheated broiler for about 10
    minutes, or until the skin is nicely charred. Transfer
    into a covered container, set aside to cool. Peel off the
    skin from the roasted peppers.
2. Put the roasted peppers and tomatoes in a food
    processor, pulse into a mixture with coarse texture.
3. Transfer into a large bowl, stir in the garlic and
    gradually add in the oil while constantly stirring. Add
    in the lemon juice, cucumber, scallions and half of
    the chopped herb mixture and stir to combine.
4. Chill for at least an hour before serving. Portion
    chilled soup into individual serving bowls, top with
    crumbled cheese and herb mixture. Drizzle with olive
    oil and serve.

Lemony Egg Soup with Peas

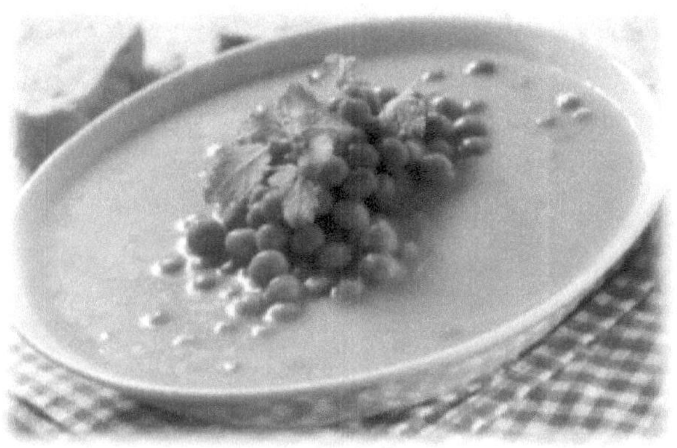

SERVES: 4 to 6

INGREDIENTS:

- 2 tablespoons of unsalted butter
- 1 shallot, minced
- 1 cup chicken broth
- 1 lemon, juiced
- 2 large eggs
- salt and coarsely ground black pepper
- 2 tablespoons of Parmigiano-Reggiano, grated
- 2 cups cooked peas

DIRECTIONS:

1. Melt the butter in pot over medium heat. Add the shallots and cook for about 2 minutes, or until soft and translucent. Add the broth and lemon juice, cover and bring to a boil. Reduce to low heat and simmer for 10 minutes.

2. While cooking the soup, add and whisk together the

eggs, salt and pepper. Gradually pour small amounts of the egg mixture in the pot, stirring constantly. Add the cheese, season with salt and pepper. Return to a simmer, remove pot from heat.

3. Portion into individual serving bowls, serve with cooked peas on top.

Mediterranean Roasted Vegetable Soup

Roasting the vegetables first brings out all their delicious sweetness. Pumpkin seeds make a lovely garnish, echoing the butternut squash in the soup.

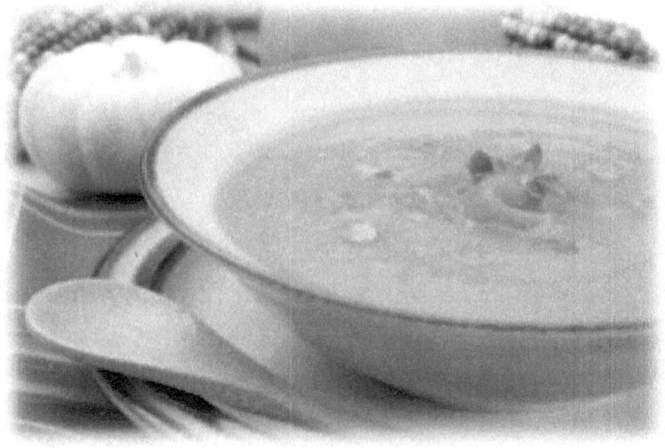

SERVES: 6

INGREDIENTS:

- 1 yellow pepper, deseeded and sliced into strips
- 1 large red onion, cut into wedges
- 1 small butternut squash, peeled and divided into 8 equal portions
- 1 red pepper, sliced into strips
- 2 large tomatoes, cut into quarters
- 1 tablespoon minced garlic
- 3 sprigs rosemary
- 1 organic lemon, juiced
- salt and freshly ground black pepper, to taste
- 2 cups vegetable stock

•

DIRECTIONS:

1. Preheat oven to 200°C. Grease a roasting tin with oil, set aside.
2. Place the vegetable on the greased roasting tin. Top with garlic, rosemary, salt and pepper, and then drizzle with lemon juice on top.
3. Roast in the oven for about 30 minutes, or until the vegetables are tender and cooked through. Discard the rosemary, set aside to cool.
4. Place half of the vegetables and the stock in a food processor. Pulse until a smooth and thick consistency is achieved.
5. Portion the remaining roasted vegetables into individual serving bowls. Reheat the pureed vegetables and pour into serving bowls. Serve warm.

LEPTIN MEDITERRANEAN HEALTHY SALAD RECIPES

There's so much more to salads than boring old iceberg lettuce and tomatoes. Use these unusual salads as side dishes, or as a light meal, perhaps accompanied by a lovely crispy crusted loaf.

Mediterranean Cucumber & Tomato Salad

SERVES: 6 to 8

INGREDIENTS:

- 2 medium cucumbers, diced
- 3 large tomatoes, diced
- 1 onion, diced or thinly sliced
- 2 tablespoons minced fresh basil
- 2 tablespoons minced fresh cilantro
- 2 tablespoons minced fresh parsley
- Salt and black pepper, to taste
- 1 organic lemon, juiced
- 4 tablespoons extra virgin olive oil

DIRECTIONS:

1. Mix together the cucumber, tomato, onion and minced herbs in a bowl. Season with salt and pepper to taste. Gently toss the ingredients to combine.
2. Cover and chill for at least 2 hours before serving.
3. Remove the bowl from the chiller and stir in the lemon juice and olive oil. Briefly toss the salad to combine.
4. Portion salad into serving bowls then serve.

Feta Salad with Pomegranate Dressing

This salad contains the "Fruit of Paradise" as pomegranate are sometimes known. They're sweet, crunchy, and brimmin with antioxidants.

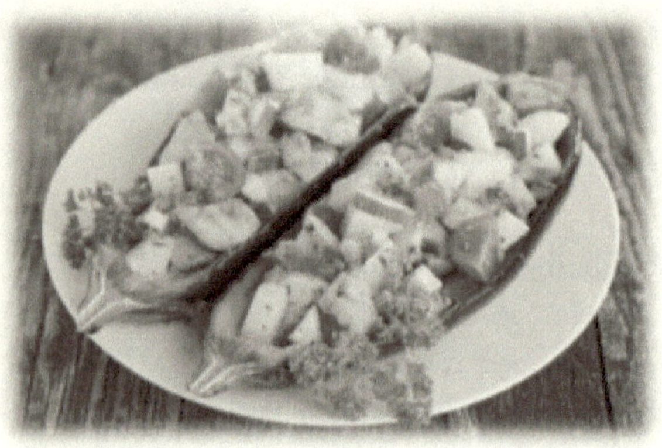

SERVES: 8

INGREDIENTS:

- 2 red bell peppers, seeded and halved/ quartered
- 3 medium aubergines, halved/quartered
- ¼ cup extra virgin olive oil
- 1 teaspoon cinnamon
- 1 cup chickpeas, blanched
- 1 red onion, halved and thinly sliced
- 1 cup feta cheese, crumbled
- ¼ cup of pomegranate seeds
- ¼ cup of fresh parsley, roughly chopped

FOR THE DRESSING:

- 2 garlic clove, minced
- 1 tablespoon lemon juice

- 2 tablespoons pomegranate molasses
- 4 tablespoons extra virgin olive oil

DIRECTIONS:

1. Preheat oven to 200°C. Place the peppers skin side up, on a greased baking sheet. On a separate greased baking sheet, place the aubergines and drizzle with olive oil. Season with cinnamon, salt and pepper.
2. Roast the peppers and the aubergines at the same time in the oven. Roast peppers for about 5 minutes, or until blackened. Transfer roasted peppers to a resealable plastic bag, set aside to cool. Scrape off the skin of the roasted peppers, discard the skin and set aside the peppers.
3. Roast aubergines for about 20 to 25 minutes until softened. Remove from the oven, set aside.
4. While roasting the vegetables, combine all ingredients for the dressing in a mixing bowl. Whisk to combine, set aside.
5. Portion aubergines into serving plates together with the greens, onions, and roasted peppers. Pour the dressing over and top with parsley. Serve.

Fig & Mozzarella salad

Just reading this recipe makes my mouth water. The combination of honey-sweet figs, crunchy hazelnuts and beans, and creamy cheese is simply stunning.

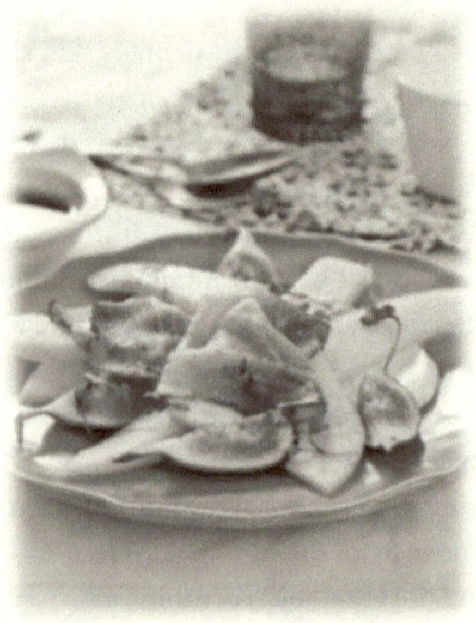

SERVES: 4

INGREDIENTS:

- 200g fine green beans, trimmed and blanched
- ½ cup fresh basil leaves, torn
- 2 tablespoons balsamic vinegar
- 6 small figs, quartered
- 1 shallot, thinly sliced
- 1 ball mozzarella, drained and diced
- ¼ cup hazelnuts, toasted and chopped
- 1 ½ tablespoons fig jam
- Salt and pepper, to taste

- 3 tablespoons extra-virgin olive oil

DIRECTIONS:

1. Portion blanched beans on individual serving plates, top off with shallots, figs, hazelnuts and basil.
2. Combine together fig jam, olive oil, balsamic vinegar in a bowl, season with salt and pepper. Whisk to combine.
3. Pour the dressing over the salad mixture and serve with cheese and extra basil on top.

Shredded Romaine and Cucumber Salad with Yogurt Dressing

This fresh green salad has a lot of flavour and looks so pretty on the plate.

SERVES: 4

INGREDIENTS:

FOR THE DRESSING:

- 2 garlic cloves, minced
- 1/2 cup Greek yogurt
- ½ organic fresh lemon, juiced
- 1 tablespoon white vinegar
- 1 to 2 teaspoons sugar
- 5 tablespoons extra-virgin olive oil
- salt and ground black pepper

FOR THE SALAD:

- 1 tablespoon chopped fresh mint
- 2 tablespoons chopped fresh flat-leaf parsley
- 1 cup of baby arugula, chopped
- ½ cup toasted walnut halves, chopped
- 2 tablespoons chopped fresh dill
- 1 large head of romaine lettuce, cut into chiffonades
- 1 cucumber, seeded and thinly sliced
- salt and ground black pepper, to taste
- ½ teaspoon red pepper flakes, crushed

DIRECTIONS:

1. In a mixing bowl, combine together the lemon juice, sugar, garlic and vinegar. Let it stand for at least 5 minutes to infuse the flavors. Whisk in the yogurt and gradually drizzle in the oil, whisking constantly to combine the ingredients. Season to taste with salt and ground pepper. Chill until ready to use.
2. Pat dry the romaine leaves with paper towels and transfer to a large bowl. Mix in the cucumbers, walnuts, dill, mint and parsley in the bowl. Chill for at least 1 hour before serving.
3. Remove the salad mixture from the chiller and toss it with the dressing. Serve with red pepper flakes and extra walnuts on top.

Shaved Fennel Salad with Toasted Almonds, Lemon, and Mint

Combining typically Mediterranean ingredients, this is another simple but beautiful dish.

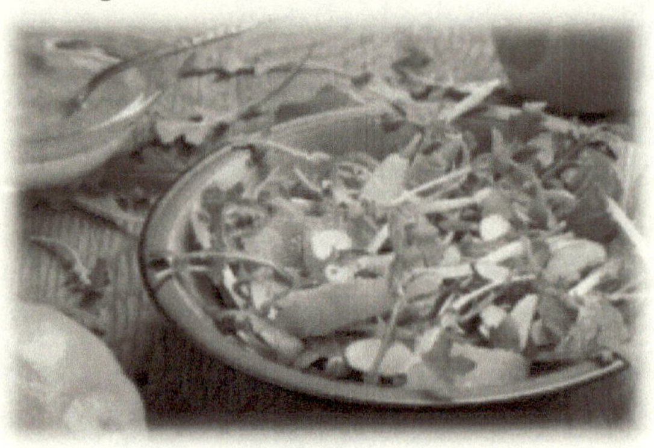

SERVES: 4 to 6

INGREDIENTS:

- 1/4 cup fresh mint leaves, torn
- 1/4 cup extra-virgin olive oil
- ½ teaspoon of coarsely ground black pepper
- 2 large fennel bulbs, trimmed and core removed
- 1 organic lemon/orange, juiced
- Kosher salt, to taste
- 1/2 cup chopped almonds, toasted

DIRECTIONS:

1. Shave the fennel crosswise with a mandolin. Place in a bowl, set aside.
2. In the bowl, toss fennel with lemon juice and salt. Let it stand for 10 minutes to infuse the flavors. Stir in

half the almonds, mint and the olive oil, toss to combine.

3. Portion salad into individual serving plates. Top with the remaining almonds and mint, finish off with freshly cracked pepper, and then serve.

Brooklyn Grange Salad with Pickled Eggs and Idiazabal

Idiazabal is a traditional hard cheese made from raw sheep's milk, and originating in Spain.

SERVES: 6

INGREDIENTS:

- 1/2 cup toasted honey pecans
- 2 cups grated radish
- 1 medium kohlrabi, grated thinly with mandolin
- 1 garlic clove, crushed
- salt and ground black pepper, to taste
- 3 tablespoons sherry vinegar
- 1 teaspoon red pepper flakes, crushed
- 2 tablespoons minced anchovy fillets
- sea salt
- ½ cup finely grated Idiazabal or Manchego cheese
- 1 tablespoon preserved lemons, finely chopped
- ¼ cup of olive oil
- 1 tablespoons Dijon mustard
- 4 cups of baby greens, roughly chopped
- 1 cup mixed fresh herbs and edible flowers, herbs cut into chiffonades
- ½ tablespoon of finely grated organic lemon zest

•

FOR THE PICKLED EGGS:

- 5 to 6 eggs, soft boiled and shells removed
- 1 cup pickled beets, solids and liquid separated

DIRECTIONS:

1. Place the eggs in a non-reactive container and pour pickling liquid to cover. Cover the container and chill for at least one day.

2. Put 2 teaspoons of oil, garlic, lemons, anchovies, teaspoon of salt and pepper in a mortar. Grind the mixture into a paste with a pestle. Transfer the paste to a mixing bowl and mix in the vinegar and mustard. Gradually stir in the oil, season with salt and pepper. Set aside.

3. In a separate bowl, add in the radishes, kohlrabi, pecans, greens, chopped herbs and mixed flowers. Adjust taste with pepper and salt. Gently toss ingredients with vinaigrette, place into a serving dish. Set aside.

4. Remove eggs and transfer into a colander, drain liquid and pat dry with paper towels. Slice the eggs into halves and place it over the salad mixture. Top with cheese, horseradish and grated zest of lemon, serve.

Poached Quince Salad

Quinces lend a lovely sweetness to this salad, and contrast well with the bitterness of the arugula and the saltiness of the ham.

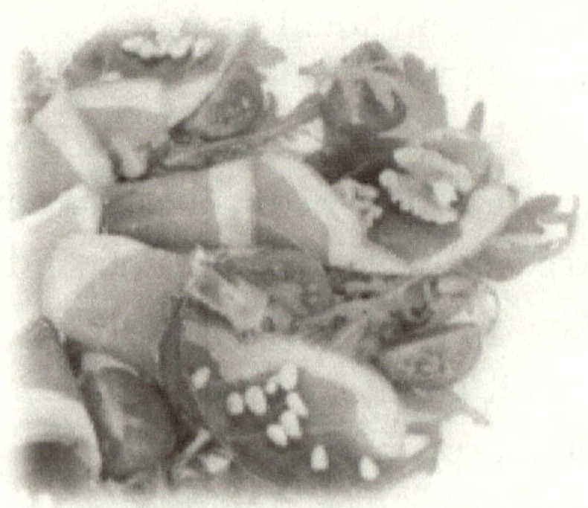

SERVES: 4

INGREDIENTS:

- 2 cups quinces, peeled and core removed, quartered
- 2 to 3 tablespoons of local honey
- Zest of 1/2 lemon, sliced into strips

- 4 cups baby arugula
- ½ cup Serrano ham or prosciutto ham, thinly sliced
- 2 Tbs. extra-virgin olive oil
- Kosher salt, to taste
- Black pepper, freshly ground to taste
- ¼ cup almonds, toasted and chopped
- ¼ cup firm Manchego or Asiago, or other mild-flavored cheeses, shaved
- 4 balsamic vinegar, preferably aged 12 to 25 years

DIRECTIONS:

1. Place the quartered quinces, organic zest of lemon and 3 tablespoons of local honey in a pan. Pour water to cover the quinces with 1 inch. Apply medium-high heat, bring to a boil and then cover with lid. Reduce to low heat and simmer for about 40 to 45 minutes. The quinces are ready when it is soft and tender. Remove from heat, set aside to cool.

2. Toss in arugula, the ham, in a mixing bowl and stir in the oil. Adjust seasoning with salt and ground black pepper. Portion the salad among serving plates. Add the quinces over the salad plates. Top off with shaved Manchego cheese and chopped almonds, drizzle salad with balsamic vinegar. Serve.

Farro Salad with Marinated Artichokes, Watercress, and Feta

Farro is a nutty, chewy grain once it's cooked, that was use by the ancient Romans.

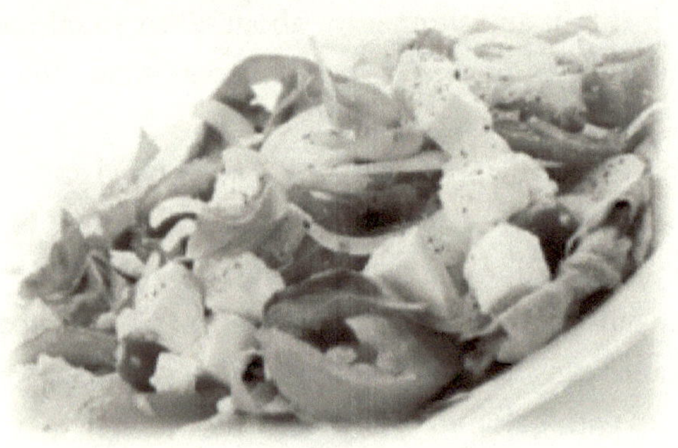

SERVES: 4

INGREDIENTS:

FOR THE ARTICHOKES:

- 2 tablespoons fresh oregano
- 1 1/2 cups extra-virgin olive oil, or as needed
- 1/2 cup white wine vinegar
- ½ cup fresh parsley
- ¼ cup fresh thyme
- 2 garlic cloves, peeled and crushed
- salt
- 4 artichokes, trimmed, and quartered

FOR THE SALAD:

- salt
- 1 cup farro

- 1 cup Feta cheese or goat's cheese
- 2 medium scallions, cut into bias
- ½ cup watercress, trimmed and chopped
- 2 teaspoons red wine vinegar
- Freshly cracked black pepper

DIRECTIONS:

1. Add 1 cup water, garlic, salt, vinegar in a pot over high heat and bring to a boil. Add the artichokes and cook until tender, or for about 10 minutes. Remove artichokes from pot and drain, pat dry with paper towels. Transfer in a bowl and add in the garlic, parsley, thyme, oregano and pour over the oil. Set aside and let it sit for about 1 hour.

2. Drain the artichokes and reserve ¼ cup of oil, discard garlic and herbs. Return artichokes and reserved oil in the bowl.

3. In a pan with salted boiling water, add and cook the faro for about 20 to 25 minutes. Drain and place on a baking sheet to cool.

4. Mix in cooked farro in the bowl with artichokes and oil. Let it rest for about 10 minutes to infuse the flavors. Mix in watercress and vinegar, season with salt and pepper to taste. Serve.

Grilled Eggplant Salad with Feta, Pine Nuts & Garlicky Yogurt Dressing

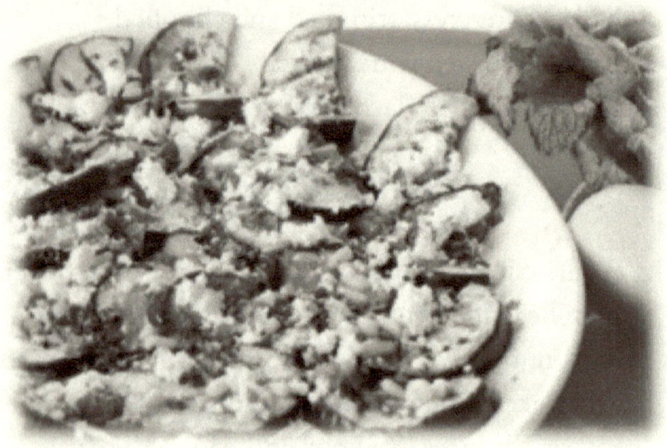

SERVES: 4

INGREDIENTS:

- 2 heads of romaine lettuce, leaves separated
- 1 large eggplant , halved and sliced
- 4 tablespoons extra-virgin olive oil
- ½ cup Greek yogurt
- ½ organic lemon, juiced
- 2 cloves of garlic, mashed into paste
- A pinch of ground cumin
- ½ cup fresh flat-leaf parsley leaves, minced
- ½ cup Feta cheese or goat's cheese, crumbled
- ¼ cup pine nuts, toasted

DIRECTIONS:

1. Place lettuce leaves in a bowl and cover with paper towels, chill.

2. Preheat gas grill with high heat, brush eggplant with 2 tablespoons of oil and season with salt and pepper. Reduce gas grill to low heat and grill the eggplant for about 3 minutes on each side. Flip to cook the other side, cook for 3 minutes. Remove from grill and transfer to a plate.

3. Remove lettuce from the chiller and portion into individual serving plates, top with grilled eggplant, feta and nuts then drizzle with dressing on top.

Tomato Salad with Feta, Olives & Mint

Similar to a traditional Greek salad, but the addition of mint and lemon freshens and lightens it.

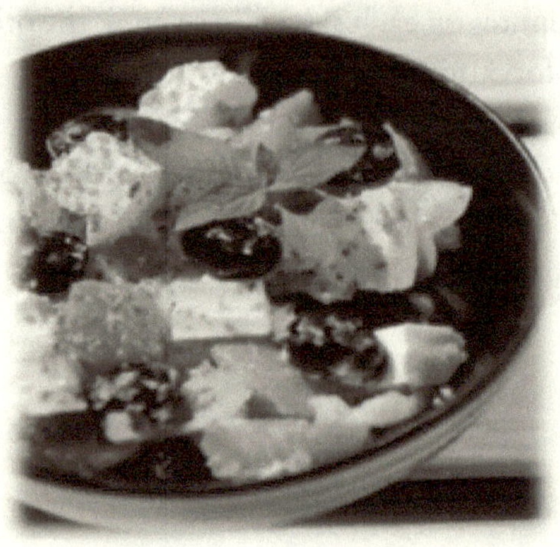

SERVES: 6

INGREDIENTS:

- 1 cup Feta cheese, crumbled
- 1/4 cup fresh mint, chopped
- 4 ripe red tomatoes, sliced into thin rounds
- Kosher salt
- 2 medium cucumber, peeled and seeded, diced
- 1 cup cherry tomatoes, halved
- 1/2 cup Kalamata olives, pitted and halved
- 4 tablespoons extra virgin olive oil
- ½ tablespoon grated organic lemon zest
- 1 tablespoon fresh organic lemon juice
- Freshly cracked black pepper

DIRECTIONS:

1. In a mixing bowl, combine cheese and mint and set aside.
2. Sprinkle with salt and pepper over the tomato slices and arrange them on a serving platter. Add the cucumbers and olives on top and chill.
3. Whisk together the oil, lemon juice and zest, salt and pepper in a bowl. Drizzle mixture over the salad and top with cheese. Serve immediately.

Conclusion

For us, it's so inspiring that eating means sharing. The coming together of friends and family to share a meal is one of the most powerful and intimate forms of communication that there is. Mealtimes should always be special occasions, richly blessed with togetherness, light-hearted conversation, and wonderful health-giving ingredients. Food for family and friends is less about spending hours in the kitchen, and more about simply opening the door to those you love and offering to share what you have.

Mediterranean principles teach us that the best meals are often the simplest, provided they are prepared with respect for good ingredients and plenty of care. So you may only have simple salad and a loaf of crusty bread, but when offered with generosity and a spirit of hospitality, they become a feast fit for royalty.

We trust that these recipes will become well-used and well-loved in your household, and that you will have as much fun making them as we have had putting them together.